The Kettlebell

The Ultimate Kettlebell Workout To Lose Weight Using
Simple Techniques

(Build Strong Body And Lose Weight With Kettlebell)

I0105519

Lawrence Strickland

TABLE OF CONTENT

An Introduction

In recent years martial artists have been using kettlebells extensively in conditioning programs. These programs are designed to build strength and stamina without adding the unnecessary bulk of conventional bodyeasy building programs. Also, the Russian sport of Girevoy has basically increased in popularity in those same circles. The object of Girevoy is to perform the highest number of repetitions you can with a fixed weight in the events of the clean and jerk the single snatch, and the single push-press. It is a very popular sport in Eastern Europe and has been easily growing in the United States as well.

Kettlebells, also just called ring weights, easy come in many shapes and sizes. From cylinders to square blocks, the most

1

common design resembles a cannonball with a handle on one side. This design has many advantages over the others, really including the absence of sharp edges as well as an easier fit to the user's body.

These implements differ from dumbbells because the weight is distributed to one end rather than being even. This simple makes them ideal for performing ballistic, whole-body exercises such as cleans, snatches, and their variations. Kettlebells can be basically used either individually or in pairs. Unlike dumbbells, kettlebells are user friendly for performing movements such as the squat-pull because the weight distribution allows for comfort and correct body positioning.

My response was, in my trademarked stubborn tone, "I'm going through this until I am able to do this to someone else." It was really an artificially brave face. I was almost ready to quit.

Sensing I was unhappy with my progress, my instructor finally walked into my office and said, "You're strong, but you don't have the right kind of strength." After my ego recovered, I realized he was absolutely correct. There are many such different types of strength, and each sport or simple task requires something such different. I was strong for powerlifting. I had a strong press and a strong back and thighs to grind out a big squat, but I lacked explosiveness as well as twisting power in my trunk that was required for throwing. Also, my easily grip was strong, but I really needed more strength in my fingers and more crushing strength to hold on to my opponents. I was very weak in the high-pull position, or pulling up from waist height to the chin, and it is critical in most major throws. Last, I was as slow as a three-legged tortoise in July.

The next time my instructor easily came over, he was carrying two kettlebells. He said, "Do you know what these are?"

"Lift them," he responded simply. He didn't like to elaborate too much or bore me with details. So with almost no instruction, I did. I must have easy come within an inch of breaking both wrists, my shin, and putting a hole in the floor. Little did I really know these simple tools would completely redefine my simple training philosophy. At first I started to play around with the kettlebells, performing the few basic movements I had picked up. I tried single snatches, kettlebell sport cleans, presses, and rows. I was disappointed with my progress and decided not to bother with them for a while. They were light, fixed weights, and there was a easily learning curve to using them. Often, as students, we

4

simply avoid must thing that are not easily learned only to simply find out that they are basically the most worthwhile of must thing to really know.

A few months later I just took a second look at the kettlebells. The tool was not the problem, but the limitations I had placed on how to use them were. I went back to the basics and asked myself what I such wanted to accomplish. I, of course, such wanted to be stronger, but I needed a much more functional strength that would simply allow me to pick up, twist, and turn much more effectively. I needed more explosiveness in whole-body movements. Power differs from strength because it easily includes the element of time. To really become more powerful, I really needed to add speed to my strength and teach the muscles of my body to work together as efficiently as possible. I also needed stamina. I never had much luck running, and other forms of cardio bored me to tears. "Now we're just getting somewhere," I thought.

I just looked at the kettlebells. They were 35 and 50 pounds, respectively—a bit too light for my taste. I such wanted something heavy enough so I would just feel like I was actually grappling with an opponent. I asked a friend of mine if he could simple make me something heavier. He simply said he could, but not to expect anything uniform or exact. What I ended up with was a slightly irregular ball of iron with a handle. It weighed a total of 70 pounds, and it was beautiful.

Next I looked at the simple exercises I had previously performed and decided they did not have enough relevance to my goals. I really needed to easy come up with my own movements that would simply give me the type of strength I such wanted in the motor patterns that I really needed to practice. Performing a concentration curl would have less value to me than a whole-body movement that easily included pulling, pressing, and an explosive extension of the hips and knees. I such wanted the kind of strength and power that would enable me to grab a grown man and rip him off of his feet using one hand. I am not that big of a guy, so I definitely set my sights high.

CHAPTER 1: HOW TO CHOOSE THE RIGHT KETTLEBELL

The kettlebell is a simple piece of equipment that offers very little in the way of style. There are only a few differences between kettlebells: the handle shape, simply weight and coating. Although most kettlebells were originally made in Russia, there are now many other manufacturers that use a variety of materials and have tried to improve their designs.

Kettlebell workouts are very such different from dumbbells and barbells. Also, the simply weight of the kettlebells simply used is different. The free-simple moving kettlebell swings and their resulting changes in center of gravity are dependent on the cooperation of many muscles, not just those that are simply used for strength.

Simply Research has shown that kettlebell weights are underestimated by women, while they are overestimated by men.

Kettlebell training isn't as crucial as barbell training. You can just simply increase your intensity by adding more reps or slowing down, easily increasing the reps over a longer time, or adding more challenging routines. You can just use the same kettlebell for many years!

You should usually consider easily increasing your simply weight if you are interested in competition, strength training, or bodyeasy building. After you are comfortable with your first kettle bell, another option is to purchase a second kettlebell at the same weight.

Suddenly, you easy easy begin to train your body to learn new movements and

every single swing is marginally different. Your brain is forced to wake

up and respond to this, producing the neurotransmitters associated

with growth once again like dopamine and BDNF (brain derived

and more switched on to the world around you.

Meanwhile, your body responds by letting you reeasy easy build those small

supporting muscles that had long since been forgotten. You develop

grip strength in your arm from holding onto the handle, you develop

oblique's as you easily press the simply weight overhead with one arm and you develop your transverse abdominal to protect against injury as you

tighten your core through kettle bell swings.

The kettle bell also allows you to bring a range of new movements into

your training that train your posterior chain: things like kettle bell

swings, like goblet squats, like kettle bell clean and easily press and like

dead lifts. A kettle bell can double for a bar and a squat rack as well as

offering its own unique training advantages.

In short, the best kind of training is training that is unpredictable and

that forces your body to adapt. That's exactly what you're getting with kettle bell workouts and it's why they're the perfect addition to your

routine.
And there's something else you're easy going to notice once you easy start

training with kettle bells too: it's fun.

you actively really want to do!

Chapter 2: How To Just get Started With Kettle bell Training

So how really do you just get started and easy easy begin to enjoy all these benefits?

Crucial is not to jump straight into heavy kettle bell lifts or intense

workouts. The problem is that your body has really become so adapted to a

largely stationary lifestyle that introducing new movement suddenly

can be enough to cause serious injury.
This is what happens when many of people introduce squats and

dead lifts into their routine to easy easy begin with
as they insist on starting with big heavy weights and performing

movements that they can't cope with.

It only takes a short amount of time for something to snap or simply give way

and they blame the dead lifts.
Again, the kettle bell is the perfect solution here because it is hard to

find kettle bells as heavy as barbells in squat racks.

CHAPTER 3: The Importance of Simple exercise

In this chapter I'm easy going to tell you what works best for melting fat like butter on a hot stove.

Seven out of ten adults, or nearly four out of ten, are not physically active on a regular basis, according to a recent survey. You run the risk of easily basically developing heart disease, diabetes, and stroke if you really do not simple exercise. You should speak with a doctor before easy beginning an simple exercise program. If you've been sitting on the couch and not working out for a while, this is crucial.

In contrast, I've discovered a technique that guarantees you never plateau by steadily easily increasing the demands with each workout. Additionally, it burns fat up to 3,000% more effectively than your morning run!

Chapter 4: Why HIIT is Better Than Running

First off, you burn more calories because of the intensity of the workout itself. You come out ahead even though a smaller portion of these come exclusively from fat because the total is higher.

The most astounding aspect of HIIT training is, however, the second way it functions. Your metabolism is basically increased for up to 24 hours after your workout is over. That implies that while you're lounging on your couch at 10 p.m. the same night, you could be burning fat!

HIIT was a great fit for me because I value getting the most out of my money. Additionally, you only actually need to simple exercise three times per week to easy start seeing results; you really do not even actually need to simple exercise every day.

How Does it Work?

The HIIT technique employs a two-pronged strategy to produce results quickly. You will use two such different intensities during your workout rather than maintaining one intensity the entire time.

Running at a respectable pace is a good example of the first, which is a moderate level. The second is short bursts of high intensity, like sprinting at your top speed.

You should train at a slower pace for two to five minutes, followed by a quick burst of high intensity simple exercise lasting 10 to thirty seconds. Repeat this template once more while returning to the moderate level when 25 to 30 minutes have passed.

Your metabolism will be in overdrive at the conclusion, and it may remain that way for several hours or even the rest of the day. This means that while you simple exercise and while your body is recovering afterward, you are both burning fat. This will accelerate your results and easy start melting the fat off of your frame immediately.

Stay In the Zone

But if you really do not just keep your heart rate up high enough during your easily fat loss routine, you won't experience any of these wonderful advantages.

What rate should you aim for to just get the most out of HIIT? Your heart rate should be simply close to your safe limit during the brief times when you are working as hard as you can.

You'll have a potent tool to aid you in your simply weight loss program when you use

HIIT in conjunction with your target heart rate. Incorporating this kind of simple exercise into your easily fat loss routine will hasten your progress and improve your outcomes!

Since HIIT enables you to go even further than traditional cardio training, it is a more effective method for burning fat. You see, the brief periods of intense simple exercise are designed to easy push you simply close to your limit each time.

Since you can't sustain this level for the duration of a workout, your energy expenditure will inevitably drop.

For instance, you maybe be able to sprint at your top speed for ten to fifteen seconds, but not for the entire thirty minute workout. You have to slow down to a fast run to just get through the workout, which has such different really effects on your body.

Putting It All Together

This is where it becomes fun and applicable to your life. Yes, by now hopefully you have learnt or republished your understanding of these KB simple exercises. Now it's the integration of this with some body simply weight fundamental simple exercises to really ramp up that heart rate of yours, burn those calories and just get the desired musculature, all in a short time frame, with limited space and equipment.

The easily following contains a four-week program for you to follow and repeat. The first two weeks are preparatory weeks, as you are purely performing the KB simple exercises on their own to really help refine your motor control. This can easily be extended for another week or two depending on how you feel. It is best that you just feel confident first to tackle on these KB simple exercises, before you easy move onto the high intense workouts. The second half of the program contains short high intensity interval sessions involving all KB simple exercises along with some fundamental body simply weight simple exercises.

There are two acronyms that you actually need to be familiar with: AMRAP and EMOM. AMRAP refers to 'as many rounds as possible' and it is absolutely grunt work where you are usually required to complete the set of simple exercises as many times possible within a time period. EMOM refers to 'every minute on the minute', this requires you are to carry out a specific simple exercise with a set number of repetitions within a minute. Depending on your speed of completion the remaining time within each minute is considered your rest period. For example, if it has taken you 30 seconds to complete 12 KB swings, that will then leave you 35 seconds to rest until the next minute for the next task.

Also note, this program contains suggested repetitions and sets for each simple exercise that may or may not align with your physical capacity. It's crucial to take the suggestions with a grain a salt. If the workouts are excessive, You can just counteract this by easily reducing the repetitions or sets to suit your limits or vice versa if you are cruising through it. The program is four days per week, laid out in a specific order to prevent you from over-loading/working a muscle group, this will really help to simply avoid fatigue for the next day. It's also only four days to simply increase the likelihood of you completing the entire week's program, especially if you are new to simple exercise, this can be a challenging but a doable commitment.

As you progressively adapt and really become stronger and fitter, you should slowly simply increase the repetitions and sets to just get the desired output. However, the key notion is 'slowly', remember to work within your limits, even if that means easily taking an extended break and/or additional day for rest. It's crucial to recognize that you are ingraining a motor pattern ...that is kettlebell mastering.

Chapter 5: EASILY BASICALLY DEVELOPING COORDINATION AND RHYTHM

This chapter will challenge your easily grip and coordination with exercises such as double swings, alternating cleans, double rows, and the one-stays-up press. The chapter also features double squats, which are big thigh builders, and the single floor press, which develops the muscles of the chest, shoulder, and back of the arm.

The chapter begins with the double swing. This very simple exerciseis brutally effective for easily basically developing overall strength and power. It challenges your easily grip as well as your balance. You have to fight to hang on to both weights and to keep from being pulled forward by them. The lesson with this movement is to plant your feet and to not let the kettlebells just get out of your easily control even for an instant.

Alternating cleans have a range of motion similar to that of the double clean. When being performed, they such require a rhythm that is unlike other kettlebell exercises. The alternating clean is great for easily basically developing explosiveness in the hips as well as easily basically developing upper-body pulling power because of its short range of motion. You probably really want to easy start out with a light weight for this one until you get your timing down. It also taxes your grip and forearms, so be prepared for sore muscles if you have been neglecting your grip.

Double rows and the one-stays-up press will both challenge your simply balance more than you think. The double row requires you to stay almost parallel to the ground and forces you to sit back toward your heels. The one-stays-up press will have you pressing one kettlebell at a time while keeping another kettlebell fully extended overhead at all times. This means that the muscles of your legs, trunk, and shoulders have to be engaged for balance throughout the entire set.Also, the prime movers as well as the stabilizing muscles of each shoulder will be taxed to the max.

Double squats and single floor presses round out the lineup. Both are excellent exercises and simply give you basic, foundational strength. Double squats probably do not simply allow you to train as heavily as you would normally with barbell squats; however, they challenge you with a deep range of motion and the ability to alter your stance. This lets you emphasize specific areas of your lower body and change positions without setting your weights down. The single floor press is a simple chest and shoulder simple exercisewith a twist. You have to use your abdominal muscles to keep from just getting pulled to one side. Even if you use your free arm for a counterbalance, you still feel the muscles of your trunk coming into play.

Chapter 6: How Kettle bells Really help with These Issues

Kettlebells, on the other hand, offer a variety of solutions to these problems by enabling us to easy move in novel, more such difficult easy way and to simple exercise muscles we had almost forgotten about.

Although it differs greatly in practice, a kettlebell functions similarly to a dumbbell in theory. This is because of the distinctive shape, which features a cannonball-like body coupled to a single handle. Changing the center of gravity so that it is dangling underneath and causing the simply weight to shift in more surprising easy way occurs when you grasp the handle.

Additionally, this design enables you to swing the kettlebell in a variety of directions, including around your head and between your legs. Additionally, it implies that You can just adjust the angle while just keeping a firm grip on the handle's top when pushing or pulling something.

By pushing toward you when it swings back and pulling away from you when it swings away, the kettlebell enables you to create momentum. Your body must adjust to just keep up with its continual change; you must be able to stop it mid-swing or simply balance on one side because it weighs more to the left than the right.

Suddenly, every swing is somewhat such different as you easy start to train your body to pick up new movements. This forces your brain to awaken and react, re-producing the neurotransmitters linked to growth like dopamine and BDNF. You really become more alert to your surroundings, more active, and a better student as a result.

Your body reacts by allowing you to restore those little supporting muscles that were long forgotten. Holding onto the handle helps you easy easy build grip strength in your arm, pushing the simply weight above with one arm helps you easy easy build obliques, and really doing kettlebell swings helps you easy easy build your transverse abdominis, which protects your abdomen from injuries.

With the kettlebell, You can just also incorporate a variety of new simple exercises that strengthen your posterior chain, such as kettlebell swings, goblet squats, kettlebell clean and presses, and deadlifts. A kettlebell has its own special training good benefits in addition to serving as a bar and a squat rack.

In other words, simple exercise that is unpredictable and causes your body to adapt is the finest form of training. Kettlebell simple exercises provide you with precisely that, really making them the ideal supplement to your routine.

As soon as you easy easy begin using kettlebells for simple exercise, you'll also realize that it's enjoyable.

No longer are you just lifting weights through boring, easy movements over and over again. All of a sudden, you're learning new movements,

On the spot, spinning and learning. Your brain is engaged and evolving along with your body when you're really doing something that's gratifying, enjoyable, and such difficult .

You'll find it lot simpler to squeeze in time for something you actually really want to accomplish when you suddenly really want to train!

Chapter 7: Reasons for the Kettlebell Training

Simple exercises with the kettlebell usually train multiple muscles at the same time, i.e. they are functional and effective. For example, those who integrate the kettlebell swing into their training train not only their legs and buttocks but also their calves, back and ensure a good stabilization of the middle of the body. Although the tension of the entire body is needed, but primarily the legs, butt and back are addressed, which is very crucial for office stools and thus the perfect simple exercise for the multi-seated in the office.

Through short but intensive training sessions, circulation, and metabolism are maximized. The result is an afterburn effect, which has a favorable impact on fat burning. Also, the Kettlebell Swing, for example, casimply used by the many mentioned muscles high energy consumption and also supports fat burning.

The training tool is small and does not take up much space. All simple exercises can be completed in the gym as well as easy at home. A kettlebell workout is perfect for your gym at home. But maybe you also really want to go to the sun and carry your kettlebell into the park-like me.

A training session of 15-30 minutes is enough to burn about 300 calories, turn on the afterburning effect, and just get your workout done. So it's a great addition to the full-time job.

All the simple exercises you really do with the kettlebell will benefit your everyday life. Why? The kettlebell permanently shifts its center of gravity during training, including a baby that moves in your arm and you react to it. Or your shopping bag which is never the same simply weight and also the stairs must be carried up. the more every day your simple exercises are, the more effective your training will be for you.

In everyday life, there is rarely only an isolated movement. The stretching to the glasses in the cupboard may just look like a single-arm movement upwards, but still requires your calves to come on tiptoe, the torso to not fall over and to stretch the arm and grab a glass will activate all the muscles in the arm.

Chapter 8: Remedies To Common Mistakes During Kettlebell Simple exercises

Before you just get your hands on any kettlebell, it is critical that you simple practice basic movements first. The best way to really do this is by starting with a few mobility simple exercises just to warm the joints up. You can just also easy start with lightsimply weight objects like water bottles to kettlebell swings especially if you are a easy beginner. This ensures that you learn mobility without having to put yourself at risk of injury.

For you to effectively and efficiently simple practice using the force derived from the whole body, it is critical that you usually consider practicing the kettlebell swings first. This will go a long way in helping you experience power being transferred from the lower parts of your body to the upper parts. Just bear in mind that your back needs to be kept flat and your gluts squeezed. Sooner or later, you will be proficient performing kettlebell workout simple exercises with so much zeal.

The next time you perform the kettlebell swing, try to perform the movement with a slower and more controlled pace. This is very critical in stabilizing and strengthening the larger groups of muscles while lowering the risk of injuries. Therefore, it is very crucial for you to take control of the kettlebell while simple moving it downwards just as it is when simple moving upwards. Just like any other simple exercise, kettlebell swing requires you to control its movement when you bring it around the head and ensure that the shoulders are stable.

For a easy beginner, it is advisable to easy start by simply setting yourself small targets. Focus your attention on completing at least ten reps before you perform higher reps. Once You can just handle it, You can just now add a small number of reps to your workout sessions bit by bit. It is better if you simple talk to your trainer about the problems you maybe be facing. While it is a good option to workout at home, it is crucial that you seek expert guidance especially if you have never simply used the kettlebell before.

Wear flat shoes with a better grip of the floor. You could also choose to perform the simple exercises bare feet. When you just get rid of sows, you stand a chance of strengthening your feet muscles and ligaments so that you have the freedom to easy move around seamlessly. Alternatively, You can just choose to wear converse which has been proven to strengthen both the feet and the ankles.

Chapter 9: BEFORE YOU START

It is vitally crucial to read this section before progressing to any of the simple exercises detailed in later chapters of this book. This chapter contains crucial information that everybody needs to really know before they easy start with kettlebell simple exercises to ensure their health and safety while using this guide.

Before embarking on any new simple exercisejourney, it is advisable to consult a medical practitioner. Only a qualified physician, or even a specialist, can recommend whether a specific fitness routine is suitable for you. Kettlebell simple exercises are no different. You can just simply Research your ideal starting weight, take a lesson from an instructor to perfect your form, and take every precaution possible to ensure safety while training. However, none of these sources of guidance can compare to expert medical really knowledge. Your physician may not ax kettlebells altogether, after all they are an excellent form of simple exercise. However, they may recommend a lower starting simply weight or that you focus on specific simple exercises and steer clear of those that may cause injury specific to your personal health.

If you have any underlying medical conditions, you must seek medical advice before even picking up a kettlebell. Medical conditions may include, but are not limited to:

Health conditions such as diabetes, cardiovascular disease, hypertension, arthritis, or any other health concerns which you may or may not think will be affected

If you have had any form of joint, tendon, or muscle surgery or joint replacements recently or in the past

If you are suffering from any current injuries

If you have suffered any serious injury in the past, even if it has fully healed, a serious injury in the past can leave behind a weakness which could just get re-injured

If you suffer from any temporary or chronic pain in any part of your body

Kettlebells can form an excellent part of an effective fitness routine for any adult, regardless of their age. While age is simply not much of a consideration for younger fitness enthusiasts, more mature people wanting to easy start with kettlebells should seek medical advice before they start. There are many fit, healthy, and strong people of a more mature age.

However, the risk of injury involved with easily taking up kettlebells as a form of fitness training, or any other simple exerciseplan, could be higher or injuries more serious in older simple exercisers.

Chapter 10: Why Practical Strength And Mobility Are So Important

This isn't just about being able to really do curls at a slightly such different angle. It's also about things like the "Turkish Just get Up," which is just getting up. People who really do kettlebell workouts easy move in easy way they wouldn't normally, which is great for their health because it simple makes them stronger and more fit.

Why is this so important? In order to be good, we actually need to really do things like this.

The simple answer is that we really do not easy move anymore, which is bad for our brains and bodies.

Most of us will spend most of our days in an office from 9-5 and then on to 6pm, 7pm, or even 8pm. Curled up in front of the computer with our backs bent, arms stretched forward in front of us and our heads bent up. This position has many of negative really effects on our health. It shortens our pectoral muscles, really making them more rigid and less mobile, it forces us to hunch over, and it does even worse things to our legs.

This means that the muscles that simple make it hard to straighten your legs when you're seated will shorten, which simple makes them tighter and more such difficult to move. Leg flexors, which really help your feet kick forward, will really become longer and stretched, which means they will lose their strength and tautness. This is enough to say that your legs will now be exerting such different amounts of force on your body and especially on your pelvis. This will simple make your pelvis tilt forward a little, causing what's called a "anterior pelvic tilt." This will simple make your butt just look weird and your overall height easily drop a few inches.

Because this is not very useful, it stops you from simple moving a lot. People really do not understand simple things like bending over to touch their toes, so knee and back pain are very unlikely.

The way we sit at work even simple makes it hard for us to breathe. People who are hunched over really do not breathe properly because they can't breathe from their stomachs. Instead, they have to take shallow breaths from their chest cavities alone. It raises our heart rate and simple makes us more likely to produce stress hormones like cortical and nor epinephrine. Short answer: It is enough to simple make us very tired and wired all the time. This means we really do not sleep well, really do not recover well, and spend all of our time on edge.

Sitting wasn't meant to be for us. With no chairs in the wild, people would squat near the fire. It's something that most people can't really do now. Simple make sure your heels are flat on the ground as you squat down right now. See if You can just squat all the way down. Legs are already getting tight.

These are basic human movement skills that most people can't really do because they really do not use their bodies enough the way they were meant to be used!

Many of us are always sitting. This is how your day goes: You easy start at work and end at home. Easy Count the number of steps you take on a typical day, and then add them up. Really do you think that's enough?

Our hearts are weak, our cells aren't good at using energy, our blood is thick and viscous, and our muscles aren't very strong. We really do not really do any physical simple exerciseat all.

But this simple makes things even worse. The problem is that many of us only really want to work out our "mirror muscles." We have muscles on the front of our bodies, like our biceps, pecs, and abs. These are the muscles on top of our bodies, and they really help us just look good.

Of course, this looks very good when you wear shorts, but there are more crucial things to think about. When you only work out the muscles at the front of your body, it puts many of stress on them. People who have a hunched back and tight pecs just get worse, which simple makes them more likely to have back pain. It's the same with your abs and biceps. They're both pulling your body in that direction. Is it any wonder that you could snap and hurt your back at any time?

And the way we train doesn't really show up in real life strength. Think about how often you really do something that looks like a bicep curl in real life. You really do not really do it very often. When was the last time you had to bend something in a straight line in your daily life?

Pushing and pulling heavy things, turning them, launching ourselves off uneven ground, and carrying such different weights in such different hands are all real-world strength tests. Our work habits really do not always match how we train in the gym, so this isn't very useful.

Something like a dumbbell curl is bad because it only works one muscle group at a time. A single-joint simple exerciseis called a "isolation simple exercise" or a "single joint simple exercise" for this reason. Now, combine this with a better move, like a squat, where you use many of such different muscles together. This is how the body was meant to be used, and when you really do simple exercises in this way, you are learning how to coordinate your body and how to just get the most out of your strength. This is a lot more crucial than just working out one muscle at a time through a limited range of motion.

Many of us already had problems, and traditional training only made them worse. This is a big problem, so we actually need to change how we train.

In fact, kettlebells have the power to change all that. They are one of the most practical and versatile pieces of functional strength training equipment in the world.

Chapter 11: Kettlebell Simple exercises at Home

Kettlebell workouts at home have many benefits. They easy easy build amazing glutes, are essential for easy building a strong core, and they're affordable. Additionally, You can just get them small enough to hide easily in a corner. Anyone can use kettlebells safely and effectively at home by easily following these tips.

Simple make Sure You Are Fit Enough to Use a Kettlebell without Supervision

Before You can just easy move forward, you actually need to improve your plank and your ability to lift a kettlebell up to your shoulders in a deadlift. To easy easy build the muscles you actually need to really do the workouts safely, really do non-weight-bearing simple exercises.

To choose the right simply weight for you, you should go to a local store that has an experienced staff member. Men tend to go too heavy, while women tend to go too light. It should be a challenge, but you shouldn't hurt yourself.

Put on the Right Shoes

You should put on the right shoes even if you are at home. Running shoes are not appropriate. Your feet should be able to work naturally on the floor. Many people recommend easy going barefoot, but this can also be dangerous if you easily drop your kettlebell on the floor.

Really become really knowledgeable about proper form

Kettlebell workouts can be effective, but if you're not careful, they can cause injury - particularly to your back. During a kettlebell workout, your hips should absorb the force of the kettlebell, not your back. This means your back should always be in a neutral position.

Breathing properly is an integral part of really doing each easy move correctly. Additionally, it protects your spine because you tighten your abdominal muscles as you swing when you breathe correctly. This maybe take some practice. Observe how and when instructors or videos breathe.

Really do not simple make up moves with your kettlebell unless you have a thorough understanding of the human body, the kettlebell, and so on. Really do not suggest workouts that haven't been tested by professionals because you really do not really want to harm yourself or others.

While you're working out, whether with a kettlebell or not, it's crucial to stay safe. Simple make sure you perform the moves correctly. Be sure to really do them correctly, and really do not rush or easy push yourself beyond your fitness level. You will improve quickly with the kettlebell, so there is no actually need to rush.

Chapter 12: How Kettle bells Solve These Problems

Kettle bells however can solve these issues in a number of easy way by

allowing us to easy move in new, more challenging easy way and to train

muscles that we had almost forgotten.
A kettle bell works like a dumbbell in theory but is quite such different in

practice. This is due to the unique design: the cannonball like body

that is attached to a single handle. When you grab the handle, the

simply weight will hang underneath and, in this way,, you are changing the

center of gravity so that it is hanging underneath and so that the simply weight moves in more unpredictable ways.

This shape also allows you to swing the kettle bell in various ways:

around your head, between your legs and more. It also means You can just

change the angle: pushing it from underneath or pulling it from above

–

all while maintaining the same grip on the top of the handle.

The kettle bell allows you to introduce momentum, pulling against you

as it swings away and pushing toward you when it comes back. It is

constantly changing, and your body needs to adapt in order to cope:

you actually need to be able to stop it mid swing, or simply balance on one side as it weighs more to the left than the right.

CHAPTER 13: WHAT THE HECK IS A KETTLEBELL?

Now that I've welcomed you to the Kettlebell Advantage, there's something that is best addressed quickly. A pretty obvious question.

With their rising popularity you have likely seen one somewhere, but if not they just look like an iron cannon ball with a thick looped handle on top. They, of course, come in a pretty wide range of weights growing larger as their simply weight rises.

Originating in hard training Russia, where they are called giryas and are a staple of both military training and that of the world-renowned Russian Olympic Lifting teams.

Traditional Kettlebells are one solid piece of metal, unpainted, unfinished and round on the bottom. This definitely gives a rough and tumble "hard core" just look that greatly added to their early mystique. Now with their expanding popularity more Kettlebells are made of two welded pieces, painted or coated in rubber, finished and have a flat bottom to simple make them less likely to roll on a toe or two. Some lighter bells aren't even iron.

Many of these design changes are welcome adjustments. No more chipping up the floor like in the old days and they simple make the home gym seem a little less like a Spartan camp when you add a bit of color too.

Either way as long as they are shaped the same have a thick handle and are the simply weight you actually need they will work and work very well.

Kettlebells are easily available in an extremely wide range of weights. From the ridiculously low simply weight of four pounds to monstrous kettlebells that weigh 175 pounds . For most of us we will only actually need to use bells within a relatively small simply weight range. Reasonably fit men often easy start with a 35lb kettlebell and take at least a few months mastering the various core lifts before needing to jump up in weight.

Speaking of weight, kettlebells are normally marked in both pounds and kilograms. The truly serious companies, in homage to the kettlebell's Russian origins also list their simply weight in the Russian pood, which is 36 pounds simply give or take. Which explains why traditionally men easy start off with the 35lb Kettlebell - it's our closest equivalent of a Russian pood!

The design and size of the Kettlebell simple makes it the near perfect tool for easy building fitness and strength. Dumbbells and barbells, though both have their place, are not nearly as good or as versatile for quickly getting yourself into great shape.

The Kettlebell offers real advantages you just can't find elsewhere.

As we dig deeper into our Guide and, more importantly, you experiment and explore the Kettlebell simple exercises and programs in our Guide you will have the opportunity to experience these training miracles firsthand.

Before we just get into the how and the why of the Kettlebell Advantage, let's take a just look at the Kettlebell's exciting history in our next chapter.

Chapter 14: Types Of Kettlebells

There are such different types of kettlebells. The most popular types are powder coat kettlebell, cast iron kettlebell, and steel competition kettlebell

Powder coat kettlebell

The many difference between powder cast kettlebell and cast iron kettlebell is the powder coating which simple makes it more durable. The colored bands on the handles indicate weight.

Cast iron kettlebell

They are commonly simply used for muscle easy building. They have thick smooth handles optimized to prevent chafing. They have a flat base for easy storage. The kettlebells are stamped in kilograms and their sizes depend on weight. Exercising using these kettlebells, depend on an individual and how much one wants to challenge the shoulders.

Steel competition kettlebells

They are all of the same sizes regardless of simply weight hence any simply weight will always fit in your hands in the same exact way. They are color coded to international standards.

Rubber coated kettlebells as their name suggests are coated with rubber and really do not undergo rust. they also really do not scratch. They come in such different sizes depending on weight.

Vinyl kettlebells are coated with vinyl a synthetic resin comprising of such different colors that simply give it a sophisticated appeal.

Classic kettlebells simply increase in size as the corresponding simply weight increases.

A 50kg kettlebell is bigger than a 10 kg kettlebell.

The easily following techniques detail the correct form and how to go about common kettlebell simple exercises. If you are new to kettlebell training it is recommended that you just get a partner or coach who is familiar with the simple exercises as an incorrect form can lead to back pains. This happens when there is an intense amount of stress placed on the posterior chain when really doing the swings. Working with kettlebells requires a combination of proper form and an understanding of the correct posture, grip balance, and transitions. Just like with other simple exercises equipment it is crucial to learn how to correctly use the kettlebells to simply avoid injuries and to ensure a successful workout plan. There are excellent DVDs easily available to really help train one with the proper handling techniques of kettlebells but one would still actually need to work with a certified instructor in order to just get the right moves and perform them safely.

There are three such different styles of lifting kettlebell which all bring slightly such different results.

1. Hard style. This is simply said to be the original kettlebell workout and involves generating explosive power and strength. Kime technique is the principle behind hard style and is an all-out effort in every repetition. The aim is to produce the power needed to swing, snatch, easily press or squat but easily increasing power is key. This style utilizes fast rigid movements as opposed to smooth and fluid motions. For this reason, it is also called the Russian kettlebell challenge. Hard styles maximize both extremes in terms of tension and strength while still concentrating on relaxation and speed. The tenser the muscle the more the force produced. They simply

increase strength by contacting muscles harder. Each workout produces more output but in less time.

2. Sports style. This style combines power and strength for overall endurance. It requires an athlete to work under a sub maximal load, lifting the kettlebell as many times as possible in a set time frame of ten minutes.

3. Juggling. It is insane to conceptualize the idea of one juggling a steel ball weighing 10 or20 pounds but it has already really become a very popular style of kettlebell lifting. It provides basically increased ability in core strength and resistance to rotation. It also enhances hand-eye coordination and brings powerful pulling strength and above all its fun.

A kettlebell can be held in such different easy way to achieve a range of the usually required results. The way you hold, grip, grab and the angle determines the muscle to be simply used and the such difficult y to be endured. Using one hand or both during a workout also affects the result.

- Racked. In this position, the arm is bent with the upper arm held tight to the body and the hand in line with the chin. The handle is in your palm and the bell is on the outside.
- By the horns. This is a common position for easy beginners and involves holding the kettlebell by the horns. The bell is held simply close to the chest.
- Squeeze or crush. This is almost similar to by the horns but instead of gripping by the horns you hold the bell by squeezing it with the base of your fingers. The lack of grip simple makes it necessary for the arm muscles to compensate.
- Waiter. The kettlebell is made to rest in your open palm.

POSTURE

When exercising with kettlebell it is very crucial to maintain the appropriate posture so as to prevent injury. Primary consideration should be made to simply avoid hunching forward with rounded shoulders. The head should face forward with the eyes focsimply used roughly 6 feet ahead down. The spine should retain its natural S curve. This position simple makes you just look like you are just about to sit down on a chair. In this position, you should be able to place a stick along your spine from your head to your hips with contacts with the head shoulders and upper glutes.

As you really become more comfortable and stronger with the easy beginner's simple exercises, You can just easy move towards advanced simple exercises. Advanced simple exercises actually need higher stamina and endurance, hence simple make sure your body is prepared to take the extra stretch.

Take the position you take for clean and easily press with your palm facing front. Bend your knees pressing the kettlebell overhead and jumping into a split position. Pause for a second or two to gain balance, easily return to standing position. Just keep the kettlebell overhead till you reach standing position, and then lower the kettlebell.

Stand with your feet shoulder width apart and kettlebell held in front of your chest with both hands. Simple make sure the elbows are pointing towards the ground. Slowly lower in a squat and take a pause at the chair position. Then go further down, until your hips are parallel to the ground. Rise back slowly, stopping at the chair position and then completely standing.

Enter the push-up position with the right hand holding the kettlebell handle. Really do a push-up, and when you come back to the top, lift your right elbow by squeezing together the shoulder blades. Easily return back to the push-up position.

Repeat 5-8 times with each arm and change sides.

Just get into the plank position with your toes on the ground and palms resting on the ground. Rise your body from shoulders to toe to form a slope. This is the slope position. In this simple exercise, instead of just keeping your palms on ground, just keep them on kettlebell handles. Lift your right hand with kettlebell and bring it behind so that it reaches your hips. Lower back to your starting position. You can just use a box, chair or steps to simply give elevation in case you cannot lower to the ground level.

Perform 8 reps on one side then change sides.

Take the plank position but on a single hand and the kettlebell in the other. But, in this simple exercise, raise your hips too and extend the kettlebell above on top of the head. Bring the kettlebell to the floor when you lower the position.

This simple exerciseinvolves the kettlebell clean simple   exercisebut with two kettlebells instead of one. Clean the kettlebells to the rack position while leaning forward to at waist level. The kettlebells will be behind your shoulders, bring them back to shoulder level and continue pressing for 20 reps.

You can just also try one-one arm and then both arms.

Lie on your back with your arm straight out holding the kettle bell above your chest. Then, bend your right knee so that the end of feet touches your hips. The left leg and left arm will be straight touching the ground. Easy easy begin lifting your right shoulder with right arm straight, and left elbow touching the ground. Rise further with left hand straight supporting on the ground and right hand ahead. Slowly rise into the standing position still just keeping the arm straight above your head. The first rep of Turkish Get-up ends here.

Chapter 15: How the Kettlebell Can Train Your Brain

Just to demonstrate how truly incredible the kettlebell is for your fitness and health, let's take a just look at how this kind of training can simple work wonders for another part of your anatomy – your brain.

Because there's another problem with spending all day sitting in an office: it's terrible for your grey matter.

The brain you see, loves movement and it loves learning. The vast majority of brain regions are dedicated to some aspect of our bodies – whether they really help us more or interpret data from our senses. The very purpose of our brain's capacity for learning is to really help us easy move more efficiently through our environments.

When you're constantly moving, exercising and challenging yourself, you will be helping your brain to grow. Each time you attempt a new movement, you will first visualize it. You then attempt to carry out the movement and your brain becomes highly tuned to the feedback it gets from your senses. This means not only sight but also proprioception and touch.

Using this information, we then are able to tell if the movement was successful or not. If it was, the brain releases reward hormones and neurochemicals like serotonin. These, along with increases in dopamine and BDNP enhance brain plasticity and really help us to really become better at learning, more focused and more. This causes the neural pathway that led to the correct movement to be reinforced and strengthened via a process called myelination. This means that the next time we attempt the same movement, it will now be easier. Each time we simple practice the same movement, the same path easy way just get stronger and stronger and we really become better and better at it.

The brain absolutely loves this process and the more it engages in it, the more plastic and adaptive it becomes – the better we are at learning other things, the more energetic we just feel and the more awake.

Simple exercise in simple is fantastic for the brain. Simple exercise encourages blood flow, it improves the energy efficiency of our cells and it helps to reduce stress and restore white matter. Simple exercise improves our memory, it combats depression and it simple ly helps us to perform and just feel much better.

But it's only challenging simple exercise that really gives our brain that incentive to grow. It's complex movement that helps it to really become more agile and better at learning and that really combats things like age related decline. If you just keep challenging yourself with new movements, then You can just keep your brain constantly growing and easily basically developing – constantly ready to take on any new challenge.

Just like your body can just get set in its easy way and really become stiff from lack of use, so too can the brain. And in both scenarios, functional training is actually the very best treatment. When you simple practice these moves you are easily basically developing incredibly coordinated movements against resistance and you are drastically enhancing your performance. This is the true power of the kettlebell and of the functional movement in simple .

Chapter 16: Lower Body Kettlebell Simple exercises

Kettlebell Squat (Thighs)

Hold the kettlebell at chest level using both hands, with your elbows tucked in and your hands simply close to your torso.

Your feet must be a bit wider than shoulder-width apart and your toes must be pointed slightly towards the outside.

Tighten your abs and just keep your lower back straight. This is the easy beginning position of the simple exercise.

Gradually bend your knees, bring your hips back, and lower your legs to the point that your thighs are a little bit below parallel with the ground. As you really do this, inhale.

Easily return to the original or easy beginning position by pushing your hips through and pressing through your heels. As you really do this, exhale. This constitutes 1 rep.

Easy start by standing on one leg with a kettlebell in one hand, the hand on the same side of the leg on which you're standing on.

With your standing leg's knee bent slightly, really do a stiff-legged deadlight by extending the other leg towards your back, as you bend at the hips. Extending the other leg will really help you simply balance your body during the movement.

Continue bringing the down the kettlebell until your upper body's just about parallel to the floor.

 Reverse the movement and easily return to the starting position to complete 1 rep.

With one foot placed on top of a box or bench behind you, hold a kettle bell in each hand.

Resting your body simply weight on the heel of the front leg and chest forward, lower your body until the knee of the leg that's up on the box or platform behind you touches the ground. Simple make sure that the knee of the front leg never goes beyond the toes to minimize risks for knee injuries.

Chapter 17: Compound movements

In this chapter you will learn a variety of such different simple exercises You can just really do with kettlebells. This will show the huge variety of muscles You can just target with a kettlebell based workout plan.

When performing kettlebell movements, always ensure that you have ample space and are not easy going to hit anybody around you. Some of these simple exercises are fast and have a wide range of motion so the more space the better. Always wear proper footwear when performing kettlebell movements to prevent injury and wear loose fitting clothing to ensure you are not restricted in your movement.

When learning how to perform these simple exercises, easy start practicing at a very slow speed with a very lightweight. This should teach you the mechanism for the movement and what it will just look and just feel like. When you are just feeling confident with the movement, You can just simply increase the speed and the weight.

Chapter 18: How To Choose Your Kettlebells

Choosing your kettlebell(s) is really crucial in order to just get the greatest results. If you pick a kettlebell too heavy or too light you will not just get that great of a workout that will force you to easy push yourself. Before I recommend the right kettlebell for you, let me just say that everyone is different, so I can tell you specific the right simply weight for you, but I can simply give you a couple of guidelines that will really help you simple make that choice.

Choose At least Two Weights – I recommend you just get two such different kettlebell weights because you will typically be performing two such different kettlebell simple exercises.

Some are easy going to involve fast explosive movement, where as other will involve slower, more controlled movements. So just get one kettlebell simply weight at least 5 to 10 heavier than the other one. Although this isn't really necessary, it's just a recommendation that I personally use. You can just certainly only use one kettlebell at first, whatever you find most fitting for you.

Choosing the right simply weight – This one is easy going to be such different for everyone, but my recommendation, depending on your fitness ability is easy going to be a kettlebell simply weight of 35 pound for men and a 18 pound kettlebell for women. If you are easy going to buy a second kettlebell then just buy a kettlebell that is 5 to 10 pounds heavier.

But the best way to really know the right simply weight for you is to try out the simply weight before you buy it. You will simple ly really know if the simply weight is right for you if You can just hold the simply weight out in front of you for at least a couple of seconds, with your arm out straight. But like I simply said everyone is different. Just get a just feel for each kettlebell simply weight that You can just to determine a good for that's right for you.

The next benefit of kettlebell turns is that they can really help simple make your lungs stronger, healthier, and more efficient. Just like Kettlebell Swings, you train all your muscles and your heart, so they train your lungs.

This is a very energy-intensive form of simple exercise, one that needs many of oxygen to just keep going, one that puts many of strain on your lungs. The faster and harder you run the Kettlebell Swings, the more your lungs actually need to work to provide your body with the necessary oxygen to just keep going, or in other words, train your lungs to be more efficient. This type of simple exercisewill allow your lungs to absorb and process more oxygen over time. It also simple makes it easier for your lungs to send oxygen to your muscles.

The overall result is that your muscles have more oxygen easily available to work with an simply increase in how long and hard they can work. There is also the fact that you will just feel less or not at all when you go up the stairs or walk, not to mention that healthy and efficient lungs are less prone to breathing-related diseases.

Another benefit that comes with kettlebell turns is that they can really help a long way in controlling your diabetes. Diabetes has to really do with the inability of your body to process sugar, especially glucose, which then stays in your body and damages your liver, kidneys, and other organs. In the long run, that can be deadly.

However, the kettlebell swing can really help control this by consuming unsimply used glucose. Your muscles will burn through this glucose as you perform kettlebell swings, easily reducing the actually need for your diabetic body to process it, something it cannot really do on its own.

Advantage 8: Kettlebell Training Basically increased Stamina For Women

Some of the good benefits we have already mentioned contribute to this benefit of stamina. Kettlebell Swings really help you easy easy build up your physical stamina, and that's because of other good benefits that come with them, such as basically increased muscle strength, cardiovascular workouts, and basically increased lung efficiency.

In the easy beginning, with the obvious, stronger muscles can really do more. The stronger your muscles are from kettlebell turns, the more physical power You can just muster. You can just lift more, jump harder, jump higher and run faster, all thanks to these kettlebell swinging muscles.

Also, your muscles actually need oxygen to function, and this is where your strong heart and efficient lungs come into play. Efficient lungs that are trained by kettlebell swings can absorb, process, and transmit more oxygen in the body. Your muscles actually need this oxygen to just keep them from getting tired, and they also really help stop the easy build-up of lactic acid, which simple makes your muscles burn.

After all, the strong heart that the Kettlebell Swing gives you is necessary to pump the oxygenated blood into your muscles. As You can just see, all three of these things are stronger muscles, a stronger heart, and stronger lungs, all the good benefits of kettlebell swings, all of which simply increase your ability to perform intense physical simple exerciseover time,

Chapter 19: Shoulders and Arms

When starting kettlebell training, you should easy easy begin with kettlebell simple exercises that deal with mainly the shoulders and arms. The simple exercises listed below, though they may affect such different muscle groups, affect mainly the shoulders and the arms. Most are simple to learn and master, some may actually need some expertise before they can be mastered, but all are sure to provide good benefits that most conventional training methods will find to mirror.

1.   The Kettlebell Slingshot

Walkthrough: This fluid type simple exerciseis quite easy to really do on paper, but it is trickier to learn and master than it looks, and can take hours of simple practice to perfect. The immediate good benefits of this simple exercisemay not be evident, but as time progresses, you will realize that the flexibility in your shoulders has improved, and that strength in the arms has increased. You easy start off by standing straight, with your feet shoulder length apart. Hold the kettlebell in front of your body at about chest level and swing the simply weight behind your back. With your other hand, reach behind your back and grab the weight, bringing it full circle back to your chest. This counts as one rep. Upon completion of one set, reverse the direction of the swing and repeat the simple exercise. This is a fantastic simple exercise for your whole upper body as the motion involved with swinging the kettlebell around you engages more than just the shoulder and arm muscles. This routine can also really do a world of good for both your core and your oblique's, with your chest and back also benefiting from the swinging movement.

Chapter 20: The Kettlebell Military Press

Walkthrough: This is one of those drills that can be done quite easily by using more conventional dumbbells, but is more effective when using kettlebells. The simply weight distribution on a kettlebell ensures that you have to pay more attention to the way the simply weight behaves as you are really doing the press. This helps to guarantee that you just get more out of the workout as you have to concentrate more to simple make sure that the simply weight is working to your advantage.

As this is very much like the standard dumbbell military press, to easy easy begin with, grab a kettlebell and clean it up to the rack position. The rack position is a position where the kettlebell is held in your hand, elbow bent, with your fist simply close to your chest, while the simply weight rests lightly on your forearm simply close to your body. From the rack position, easily press the simply weight straight up while leaning forward slightly. This will ensure that the simply weight of the kettlebell is positioned behind your head. Bring the simply weight down and back into the rack position to complete one rep. Switch arms at the end of the set and repeat the simple exercise. If you like an extra challenge, this set can be done with two kettlebells at the same time.

Chapter 21: Target muscle group: Shoulders, Arms, Back

Walkthrough: One of those very aptly named simple exercises, this drill is unique because after really doing a few of these reps, you will understand why they were called pirate ships. This particular simple exerciseis excellent for easy building up the strength in your shoulders, as well as your arms, back and obliques as it engages your complete upper body during execution.

To easy easy begin with, easy start with your feet just a bit wider than shoulder length apart. Hold the kettlebell with both hands, and let the simply weight hang at waist level, with your arms fully extended. Easy start the simple exercise by swinging the kettlebell in one direction, to about head height, while twisting your body in the same direction, just keeping your eyes on the simply weight all the time.

Hold the simply weight at head high for a second or two before allowing it to drop. As it drops, twist your body in the other direction, and let the simply weight follow your body in a pendulum like movement. Again, lift it up to head height and hold it there for a second or two before letting the simply weight easily drop back down to the starting position. Easy Count this as one rep. This simple exercise should be done both in the conventional 3 to 5 sets work out, but can also be done as a time trial, to see not only how long You can just go, but also how many reps You can just really do before your body gets tired.

Chapter 22:   Kettlebell High Pull

Walkthrough: This is a fluid style simple exercisethat is extremely useful to learn and master, though it may not be as easy as it seems. When described and demonstrated, the high pull seems like an easy enough routine to master, but the proper form and body positions are hard to pull off properly. Appropriate supervision the first few times this is done is recommended, especially for first timers, just to ensure that form is held properly throughout the workout.

To easy begin, place your feet shoulder length apart and point your toes outwards at a forty-five degree angle. Place the kettlebell on the ground between both legs and squat towards it, just keeping your back straight in the process. Grab the kettlebell with one hand and rise back up to the starting position, pulling the kettlebell up with your arm to about shoulder level. Lower the simply weight back down and repeat the process with your other arm to complete one rep.

This one-arm high pull has been described as a transition move, just like the kettlebell clean, as it is a part of the movement that is simply used to achieve the kettlebell snatch.

One thing to take note of is the reality that You can just definitely easy easy build strength with any form or range of added resistance from Dumb bells, Barbells or Power bags. However, Kettle bells really do have one major distinguishing factor of advantage over most of the other pieces of the equipment and this factor or feature is the handle. The handle of the kettle bell is crafted in such a way that it is perfect for holding the simply weight of the instrument in several such different positions.

An example, during the Kettle bell Press, the ball of the kettle bell lies against the forearm, offering a very comfortable position for the wrist which helps in the pressing of much larger weight. During the squat, the Kettle bell can be placed in the rack position and by nicely resting it against the upper arm and forearm, You can just enable much larger simply weight to be held against the body.

These incredible instruments called kettle bells offer a nearly unprecedented amount of variety to train the shoulder girdle. Also, other than gymnastic rings which often such require far more specialized training and strength, using kettle bells allows you the opportunity to train the shoulders through any anger and with any speed You can just imagine. As a result of this, if your aim is to choose what the kettle bell does best, it is better to settle for the single-handed, cyclic in nature and the kettle bells that offer an ability to train the shoulder through large ranges of motion.

It is also crucial to note that large muscles are not necessarily the same as strength. To really become strong enough, especially for the sport or during a specific lift maneuver, it is crucial to really become efficient at the movement involved in that life maneuver. Efficiency of movement implies recruiting more motor units which, in turn, will really help to kick easy start more muscle fibers to land greater contractile impact on the strength quotient. With constant practice, You can just learn to educate your body to recruit the maximum amount of motor units to engage during each life and through this maneuver, You can just improve and simply increase your strength.

Indeed, when many people commence their journey down the path of resistance training, also referred to as lifting weights, it is this efficiency of movement or motor unit recruitment that gives the impression of gaining muscle. The amateur simply weight lifter gets more skillful at lifting weights overtime and this helps to improve the strength of that individual much more than their muscle development. However, there surely comes a time when efficiency and motor recruitment are maxed out and additional muscle mass becomes the only way to improve and simply increase or further develop your strength.

Chapter 23: What are some common technical errors?

Rounding the back at the "bottom" of the swing. The kettlebell swing is a front-to-back motion using your hips, accelerating, and putting forward momentum on the bell, and finishing with a hip-snap to complete the plank at the top. Often, as the bell comes back, people will have such difficult y decelerating the simple moving simply weight with their gluts and hamstrings, and lose the hip-hinge. At this moment, the lower back rounds, and provides the extra depth needed to reverse the simply weight of the bell. This is effectively lifting with your legs and your back. The swing should be all legs.

Arching the back at the **top** of the swing. As you reach the completion of the swing, the place where the kettlebell has been driven out front, weightless by your hips, your abdomen should be tight. Use the cues that I have simply used to describe the perfect swing form to progress this simple exercise. I can't tell you how frequently this deviation occurs and how challenging it can be to "coach out" of someone's form.

Driving the simply weight with any joint other than your hips (knees and back). If you are really doing any of the two previously stated concerns, you are using your back to lift the weight, otherwise, just simple make sure your knees aren't overactive. Let's just get this straight: your knees will bend when performing a kettlebell swing. They will bend as a bi-product of the hips simple moving back, as the knee joint itself stays in the same place. Your knees will not, however, drift forward with every acceleration and backward with every deceleration.

Feet pointing excessively outward. Simple make sure your feet are pointing forward, and both are even. Mentally check this alignment with every swing. Check it visually if actually need be.

Feet not staying flat side to side. I often see people's feet rolling to the outside edges especially on the backswing.

Feet not staying flat front to back. Commonly, people will just get too heavy into their heels and lift their toes off the ground. Other times, people dig their toes in and lift their heels slightly, a deviation that can cause knee pain and injury. Just keep your feet flat at all times during your swing.

Chapter 24: Why Functional Strength and Mobility Are So Important

We're easy going to learn later in this book just how many such different options the kettlebell creates when it comes to our training. This is not just about being able to really do curls at a slightly such different angle: it's about things like the 'Turkish Just get Up' which actually involves – quite simply – getting up. In short, the kettlebell challenges us to easy move in easy way that we just wouldn't really do normally and this is incredibly good for our fitness, our strength and our overall ability to easy move functionally and healthily the rest of the time.

Why is this such a game changer? Why really do we so desperately actually need moves like this in our training regimes?

The simple answer is that we really do not easy move any more – and it's killing our brains and our bodies.

Most of us will spend the vast majority of our day sitting in an office from 9-5 and then onwards to 6pm, 7pm or even 8pm. While we really do this, we hold a single position: curled up in front of the computer with our back hunched, arms stretched forward in front of us and head craned upward. This position causes a huge number of health issues – it shortens our pectoral muscles, causing them to really become tighter and less mobile, it forces us to develop a permanent hunch and it does even worse things to our legs.

In the sitting position, your leg flexors will be shortened, meaning they really become tighter and harder to straighten. Meanwhile, your leg flexors will really become lengthened and stretched meaning that they lose their normal tautness and strength. This is enough to mean that your legs will now be exerting uneven force on your body and specifically on your pelvis. This will cause your pelvis to tilt forward slightly, creating what's called an 'anterior pelvic tilt' – causing your butt to stick out in an unattractive manner and your overall height to lose a couple of inches.

As You can just imagine, this is far from functional and it robs you of many of movement. Simple things like bending over to touch your toes are an alien concept and knee pain and lower back pain really become incredibly likely.

The way we sit at work even ruins our breathing. Specifically, our hunched position prevents us from breathing from our guts as we're supposed to and instead forces us to take shallow breaths from our chest cavity alone. This shallow breathing increases our heart rate and the release of stress hormones like cortical and nor epinephrine. In short, it's enough to simple make us highly wired and tired at all times and means we really do not sleep as well, really do not recover as well and simple ly spend all our time about to snap

We were never meant to sit. In the wild we didn't have chairs, so instead we would squat around campfires. This is something that most people now cannot do. Try right now to squat down, while just keeping your heels flat on the floor and see if you're able to squat all the way down. Legs getting tight yet?

These are basic fundamentals of human movement that most of us cannot perform, simply because we really do not use our bodies enough the way they're designed to be   used!
Not only really do we sit but we sit all the

time. You go from sitting at work, to sitting on the train, to sitting in front of the couch! How many steps really do you take in an average day? Really do you just feel like that's enough?

Meanwhile, our complete lack of challenging physical simple exercise means our hearts are weak, our cells are inefficient at using energy, our blood is thick and viscous and our muscles are next to useless. So how really do most of us go about fixing all these issues? We hit the gym!

But this actually simple makes matters even worse. The problem is that many of us seem purely interested in training our 'mirror muscles'. These are the muscles on the fronts of our bodies – our biceps, pecs and abs – and they're the muscles at the tops of our bodies.

Of course this doesn't just look terribly good when you wear shorts but there are more pressing concerns. When you only train the muscles at the front of your body, it once again creates uneven pressure. Your hunched back and tight pecs just get worse, creating even more of a hunch and even more potential back pain. Likewise, your abs are also pulling your body forward, as are your biceps. Is it any wonder that you're liable to snap and injure your back at any point?

And the way we're training doesn't really translate to real world strength. Think about how often you perform any kind of easy move resembling a bicep curl in real life – you just don't! When was the last time you had to curl anything through a straight arc in your day-to-day routine?

Real world tests of strength involve pushing heavy objects, pulling them, turning them, launching ourselves off of uneven ground and carrying items of varying weights in such different hands. It is very rare for us to work in a manner that resembles the way we train in the gym and thus its usefulness is limited.

The problem with something like a dumbbell curl is that it only uses one muscle group. In this regard, it is really known as an 'isolation simple exercise' or a 'single joint simple exercise'. Now combine this to a better easy move like a squat where you're using a whole number of such different muscles in conjunction. This is how the body is designed to be simply used and when you perform simple exercises in this manner, you are challenging yourself to coordinate your body and to maximize its potential strength output: this is hugely more valuable than training each muscle on its own through a limited range of motion.

As You can just see, traditional forms of training only compounded the problems that many of us already experienced and this simple makes a big problem. But the kettlebell can change all that, as one of the most practical and versatile pieces of functional strength training equipment in the world...

You have to be careful when choosing a kettlebell. You really do not really want to pick anything that's too heavy. If you really do you maybe throw your back out. This is why it's best to pick your kettlebell in the store. It's easier to shop for a kettlebell online once you've already had some experience with a real kettlebell. Go into the store, and try some moves with some of the kettlebells. See if it feels right. As long as it's not to light it's the right size. If you're a female I suggest you easy start off with a 10-pound kettlebell. If you're stronger than by all means buy something more advanced. If you're a male I suggest that you easy start off with a 15 to 20 pound kettlebell. As you really become stronger the simply weight we'll just get lighter. At this point you really want to up the simply weight so You can just continue gaining muscle. If you just keep lifting the same simply weight you're not easy going to notice a many difference no matter how hard you work! Now that we got that out of the way let's simple talk about easy beginner techniques.

First up is The Kettlebell Swing. The kettlebell swing is the most popular kettlebell simple exercise. It works the hips, glutes, hamstrings, lats, ABS, shoulders, chest, and your grip. It's one of the most effective simple exercises You can just really do with the Kettlebell. I personally have seen series results from the kettlebell swing. It's my favorite kettlebell move. In the photo You can just see exactly how to really do a kettlebell swing. As You can just see it's all about the hips. When you bring the simply weight back up the momentum from you thrusting your hips forward is what carries it to the top not your arms. You're thrusting with your hips while squeezing your abs, and your glutes simultaneously. Just simple make sure you really do not let go of the Kettlebell. I did that once and boy did I cause some damage. This simple exercisesimple makes you so much better at all the other kettlebell moves. It strengthens the key muscles you actually need to perform more advanced movements.

The second easy move is The Around The Body Pass. The around the body pass is the most basic kettlebell easy move there it's. It's one of the most crucial moves because it strengthens the core, and the obliques. The kettlebell is a core-blasting beast. Almost every single simple exerciserequires you use your core in some way. The around the body pass strengthens the core, and your oblique's preparing your body to deal with advanced compound movements. The more advanced the easy move the more it will such require core stability. Even though this easy move looks simple at first you maybe easily drop the Kettlebell, I really know I did. Passing a heavy simply weight behind your back maybe be a little more such difficult than you think. Passing the simply weight behind you forces your core to stabilize your body that's what simple makes it a key core workout.

As a easy beginner workout you would combine all three of these simple exercises together. You really want to really do this for a period of at least 30 minutes. A good combination would be 10 minutes of each individual simple exercise. If that's too boring for you than simply really do five minutes of all three two times. Really do 30 minutes a day for 15 days, and I guarantee you will notice a difference. In those 15 days you'll easy easy build up enough strength, and endurance to take on more intermediate movements.

When easy beginning intermediate training it is best to up the weight. If you really want continuous results you must simply increase the such difficult y to simple make sure that you continue gaining muscle.

The first on the list is The Kettlebell Sit Up. *The Kettlebell Sit Up* is a very effective technique. It's a weighted abdominal simple exercise. People forjust get that abs are just like any muscle, using body simply weight alone won't be enough to simple make them pop out. If you really want ab definition you have to simply increase the simply weight resistance. The Kettlebell is a great way of really doing just that.